I0837987

Chapter 1: Understanding Croup

What is Croup?

Croup is a common respiratory condition that primarily affects young children, characterized by a distinctive barking cough, hoarseness, and difficulty breathing. This illness typically occurs when the upper airways become inflamed, often as a result of viral infections, particularly those caused by parainfluenza viruses. While croup can be alarming for parents due to its sudden onset and the intensity of symptoms, it is usually manageable at home. Understanding the nature of croup, its causes, and its symptoms is vital for parents navigating this condition.

The symptoms of croup often begin with a cold, including a runny nose and fever, which can quickly progress to the hallmark barking cough. These symptoms are typically exacerbated at night, leading to increased anxiety for both the child and parents. In addition to the cough, other signs may include stridor, a high-pitched wheezing sound that occurs during inhalation, and respiratory distress, which can manifest as difficulty breathing or a rapid breathing rate. Recognizing these symptoms early is crucial for effective management and treatment.

Croup is frequently linked to seasonal allergies, as allergens can irritate the airways and contribute to inflammation in susceptible children. Allergic reactions can exacerbate respiratory symptoms, making it essential for parents to monitor their child's exposure to common triggers like pollen, dust mites, and pet dander, particularly during peak allergy seasons. This connection highlights the importance of a comprehensive approach to managing not only croup but also overall respiratory health in children with allergies.

Home remedies play a significant role in alleviating croup symptoms. Parents may find that using a humidifier improves breathing by adding moisture to the air, which helps soothe inflamed airways. Keeping the child calm is also essential, as stress and crying can worsen breathing difficulties. Warm fluids and cool night air can provide additional relief. However, it is important for parents to distinguish between mild croup, which can typically be managed at home, and more severe cases that may require medical intervention.

In some instances, croup can lead to recurrent respiratory issues, and parents should be aware of the potential long-term effects. Children who experience recurrent croup may have a predisposition to other respiratory illnesses or develop conditions such as asthma later in life. Understanding the nature of croup and its implications for future health can empower parents to make informed decisions about their child's care. In severe cases, emergency treatments may be necessary, including the administration of corticosteroids or nebulized epinephrine, underscoring the importance of being prepared for all scenarios.

Causes of Croup

Croup is primarily caused by viral infections, with the parainfluenza virus being the most common culprit. Other viruses, such as adenovirus, respiratory syncytial virus (RSV), and influenza, can also lead to the development of croup. These viruses typically spread through respiratory droplets when an infected person coughs or sneezes. Children, particularly those between the ages of six months and three years, are more susceptible to these infections due to their developing immune systems. Understanding the viral nature of croup is crucial for parents, as it highlights the importance of maintaining good hygiene practices to prevent the spread of germs.

Another significant factor in the onset of croup is seasonal allergies. Allergens such as pollen, dust mites, and pet dander can exacerbate respiratory issues, making children more vulnerable to viral infections that lead to croup. When children already have inflamed airways due to allergies, they are at a higher risk for developing croup symptoms after exposure to viral triggers. Parents should be aware of their child's allergy history and consider monitoring for seasonal changes that could affect their child's respiratory health.

Environmental factors also play a role in the incidence of croup. Dry air, especially during the colder months when indoor heating systems are used, can irritate the throat and airways, making it easier for viruses to cause croup. This is where humidifiers can be particularly beneficial. By adding moisture to the air, humidifiers can help soothe irritated airways and reduce the severity of croup symptoms. Parents are encouraged to use humidifiers in their child's room during peak croup seasons, as this simple home remedy can offer significant relief.

In addition to viral infections and environmental triggers, anatomy can also contribute to the risk of croup. Young children's airways are smaller and more susceptible to inflammation than those of adults. When the throat becomes inflamed due to a viral infection, it can lead to the characteristic barking cough and stridor associated with croup. Parents should keep this anatomical factor in mind, as it helps explain why certain children may experience croup more frequently than others, especially if they have a history of respiratory issues.

Finally, recurrent croup can lead to long-term effects on a child's respiratory health. Frequent episodes may indicate underlying issues such as asthma or chronic allergies, which require careful management. Parents should remain vigilant and consult healthcare providers if their child experiences recurrent bouts of croup. Recognizing the connection between croup and other respiratory conditions can guide parents in making informed decisions regarding their child's health, ensuring timely interventions and appropriate treatments when necessary.

Symptoms of Croup

Croup is characterized by a distinct set of symptoms that can be alarming for both children and parents. The most common symptom is a distinctive barking cough, which often resembles the sound of a seal. This cough can be particularly distressing and is usually more pronounced at night, making it a key indicator for parents to recognize. In addition to the barking cough, children may also experience a hoarse voice and difficulty breathing, especially during inspiration. These symptoms are the result of inflammation in the upper airways, which is typical in cases of croup.

Another significant symptom to be aware of is stridor, a high-pitched wheezing or whistling sound that occurs when a child breathes in. Stridor is often more evident when the child is agitated or crying, and it may subside when the child is calm. Parents should monitor the severity of stridor, as it indicates the level of airway obstruction. If stridor is present at rest, it may signal a more severe case of croup that requires immediate medical attention. Observing these symptoms can help parents determine the appropriate course of action.

Accompanying the respiratory symptoms, children with croup often experience fever and general malaise. These additional symptoms can help differentiate croup from other respiratory illnesses. While croup is typically caused by viral infections, such as parainfluenza, it is important for parents to understand that the presence of fever can vary. Some children may have a mild fever, while others may experience a higher temperature. Regardless, any significant fever in conjunction with respiratory distress should prompt a consultation with a healthcare provider.

It is also important for parents to recognize that croup can be exacerbated by environmental factors, especially during certain seasons when respiratory infections are more prevalent. Seasonal allergies may contribute to inflammation in the airways, making children more susceptible to croup symptoms. Parents should consider their child's allergy history and monitor for any signs of concurrent allergic reactions, as managing these allergies can be a key part of preventing and treating croup.

In severe cases, children may exhibit signs of respiratory distress, such as rapid breathing, difficulty swallowing, or lethargy. These symptoms indicate a medical emergency, and parents should seek immediate treatment. Understanding the spectrum of symptoms associated with croup can empower parents to act swiftly, whether through home remedies, natural treatments, or emergency interventions, ensuring the well-being of their child during this challenging time.

Chapter 2: The Connection Between Croup and Seasonal Allergies

How Allergies Trigger Croup Symptoms

Allergies can play a significant role in triggering croup symptoms, particularly in children who are predisposed to both conditions. Croup is characterized by inflammation of the upper airway, which leads to a distinctive barking cough, stridor, and difficulty breathing. When allergens such as pollen, dust mites, pet dander, or mold spores are inhaled, they can provoke an immune response. This response often manifests as inflammation and swelling in the airways, exacerbating the symptoms of croup, especially in children who are already sensitive to these triggers.

Seasonal allergies are particularly relevant to understanding croup, as they often coincide with periods when respiratory viruses are more prevalent. During spring and fall, when pollen counts are high, many children experience allergic rhinitis, which can further irritate the airways. This irritation can lead to increased mucus production and swelling, creating a perfect storm for the development of croup symptoms. Parents should be vigilant during these seasons and recognize the interplay between allergy season and the onset of viral infections that lead to croup.

Home remedies can be effective in managing symptoms when allergies trigger croup. Maintaining a clean environment by reducing dust and allergens can help minimize exposure. Regularly washing bedding, using air purifiers, and keeping pets out of children's bedrooms can contribute to a healthier indoor air quality. Additionally, using saline nasal sprays can help clear mucus and allergens from the nasal passages, providing relief and potentially reducing the severity of croup symptoms.

The use of humidifiers is another natural treatment that can alleviate croup symptoms triggered by allergies. Moist air can soothe inflamed airways, making breathing easier for children experiencing stridor and a barking cough. Parents should aim to maintain a humid environment, especially at night when symptoms may worsen. It is essential to keep the humidifier clean to prevent mold and bacteria growth, which could exacerbate allergic reactions and respiratory issues.

Understanding the connection between allergies and croup is crucial for effective management. Parents should be aware of their child's allergy triggers and take proactive steps to mitigate exposure. By incorporating natural treatments such as maintaining humidity levels, utilizing home remedies, and keeping allergens at bay, parents can help manage their child's symptoms more effectively. This holistic approach not only addresses the immediate symptoms of croup but also promotes overall respiratory health, reducing the likelihood of recurrent episodes.

Identifying Allergens

Identifying allergens is a crucial step for parents navigating the challenges of croup and its connection to seasonal allergies. Allergens are substances that can trigger an allergic reaction in sensitive individuals, and understanding these triggers can help manage and alleviate symptoms associated with croup. Common allergens include pollen, dust mites, mold, pet dander, and certain foods. For children with a predisposition to allergies, exposure to these irritants can exacerbate respiratory issues, including croup, leading to increased coughing, wheezing, and difficulty breathing.

To effectively identify potential allergens, parents should observe their child's symptoms in relation to specific environments or activities. Keeping a symptom diary can be beneficial, noting when symptoms worsen and the possible environmental factors at play. For example, if a child experiences heightened symptoms during particular seasons, such as spring or fall, it may indicate a pollen allergy. Alternatively, if symptoms seem more pronounced during indoor activities, dust mites or mold could be the culprits. This methodical approach allows parents to pinpoint triggers and take steps to minimize exposure.

In addition to environmental observations, allergy testing can provide valuable insights. Consulting with a healthcare professional, such as an allergist, can help determine specific allergens through skin prick tests or blood tests. Understanding a child's unique allergy profile can empower parents to create a safer home environment. For instance, if mold is identified as a trigger, addressing damp areas in the home and ensuring proper ventilation becomes essential in managing both allergies and croup symptoms.

Implementing strategies to reduce allergen exposure is vital. Parents can take proactive measures such as using air purifiers, regularly cleaning to reduce dust and dander, and using hypoallergenic bedding. In addition, maintaining a clean and organized living space can help minimize allergens that contribute to respiratory distress. Utilizing humidifiers can also aid in creating a more comfortable atmosphere, as they add moisture to the air, helping to soothe irritated airways and alleviate croup symptoms, especially during dry seasons.

Ultimately, identifying allergens is an ongoing process that requires vigilance and adaptability. Parents should remain attentive to their child's reactions and be prepared to adjust their management strategies as needed. Understanding the interplay between croup and seasonal allergies enables parents to take a proactive stance in safeguarding their child's health. With the right information and tools, it is possible to create a supportive environment that reduces the frequency and severity of croup episodes, ensuring better overall respiratory health for children.

Managing Seasonal Allergies

Managing seasonal allergies in children is crucial, especially for those who are prone to croup. Seasonal allergies can exacerbate respiratory issues, leading to increased inflammation in the airways.

Parents should be vigilant in recognizing the symptoms of allergies, which may include sneezing, nasal congestion, and itchy eyes. These symptoms can mimic or worsen the symptoms of croup, such as a barking cough and difficulty breathing. By effectively managing seasonal allergies, parents can help reduce the frequency and severity of croup episodes in their children.

One of the primary strategies for managing seasonal allergies involves minimizing exposure to allergens. Common allergens include pollen, dust mites, and pet dander. Parents can reduce indoor allergens by regularly cleaning their homes, using high-efficiency particulate air (HEPA) filters, and keeping windows closed during high pollen seasons. When outdoor allergens are at their peak, it may be beneficial for parents to limit their children's outdoor activities, especially during windy days or early morning hours when pollen counts are highest.

Home remedies can also play a significant role in alleviating allergy symptoms. Saline nasal sprays can help clear nasal passages, while warm baths can soothe irritated skin. Additionally, honey may provide relief for some children, as it has natural anti-inflammatory properties. However, parents should consult with a pediatrician before introducing any new remedies, particularly for younger children and infants, to ensure safety and appropriateness.

The role of humidifiers in managing both croup and seasonal allergies cannot be understated. Humidifiers add moisture to the air, which can help ease respiratory discomfort caused by dry air, especially during colder months when indoor heating is used. Keeping the air humid can alleviate coughing and help children breathe easier, especially during allergy season. Parents should ensure that humidifiers are maintained properly to prevent mold and bacteria growth, which can worsen respiratory symptoms.

In addition to these management strategies, it is essential for parents to understand the connection between croup and seasonal allergies. Children with a history of allergies may experience recurrent croup due to increased airway sensitivity. Being aware of this relationship can empower parents to take proactive measures, such as closely monitoring their child's allergy symptoms and seeking medical advice when necessary. By effectively managing seasonal allergies, parents can contribute to better overall respiratory health and potentially reduce the incidence of croup in their children.

Chapter 3: Viral Infections that Cause Croup

Common Viruses Responsible for Croup

Croup is primarily caused by viral infections, with several specific viruses being responsible for the condition. The most common virus linked to croup is the parainfluenza virus, particularly types 1 and 3. This virus is known for causing inflammation in the airways, leading to the characteristic barking cough and stridor associated with croup. Other viruses that can cause croup include respiratory syncytial virus (RSV), adenovirus, and influenza virus. Understanding the viral origins of croup can help parents recognize the signs more effectively and seek appropriate care when necessary.

Another notable virus is the human metapneumovirus, which has gained attention in recent years for its role in respiratory illnesses in children, including croup. This virus often presents similarly to RSV and can lead to severe respiratory symptoms, particularly in infants. Parents should be aware that the presence of these viruses in the community, especially during the fall and winter months, can increase the likelihood of croup episodes. Keeping track of seasonal patterns can help parents prepare for potential outbreaks.

While croup is predominantly viral, it is essential to consider the connection between these infections and seasonal allergies. Allergens can exacerbate the symptoms of croup, as they may cause additional inflammation in the respiratory tract. Children with a history of allergies may experience more frequent croup episodes, particularly during allergy seasons. Parents should be vigilant about managing their child's allergies, as this can help minimize the severity and frequency of croup symptoms.

When managing croup symptoms at home, natural treatments can be beneficial. Humidifiers are particularly effective in providing moisture to the air, which can soothe inflamed airways and ease breathing difficulties. Cool mist humidifiers are recommended, as they can help reduce swelling in the throat and ease the barking cough. Additionally, parents should ensure their child stays well-hydrated and consider using saline nasal sprays to relieve nasal congestion, which can also contribute to breathing problems.

In cases where a child experiences recurrent croup, it is important for parents to monitor long-term effects and consult healthcare providers for ongoing management strategies. While most children outgrow croup by the age of five, some may experience repeated episodes, which can impact their overall health and well-being. Understanding the signs of severe croup, such as persistent stridor or difficulty breathing, is crucial for timely emergency treatment. Parents should be aware of when to seek medical help, ensuring that their child receives appropriate care to prevent complications associated with severe respiratory distress.

Recognizing Viral Symptoms

Recognizing viral symptoms is essential for parents to effectively manage croup and differentiate it from other respiratory illnesses. Croup is primarily caused by viral infections, most commonly the parainfluenza virus. Parents should be vigilant in observing their child for the hallmark symptoms of croup, which include a distinctive barking cough, stridor (a high-pitched wheezing sound during breathing), and hoarseness. These symptoms often occur after a preceding upper respiratory infection, such as a cold, making it crucial for parents to monitor their child's health closely during cold and flu seasons.

In addition to the classic symptoms, parents should also be aware of signs that may indicate the severity of the condition. Mild croup may present with a cough and some difficulty breathing, while severe croup can lead to increased respiratory distress, a rapid heart rate, and cyanosis (a bluish tint to the skin). If parents observe their child struggling to breathe or exhibiting signs of distress, it is important to seek medical attention promptly. Understanding these symptoms can help parents make informed decisions about when to provide home remedies and when to pursue emergency treatment options.

Home remedies can be effective in alleviating mild symptoms of croup. Humidifiers play a vital role in easing breathing difficulties by adding moisture to the air, which can soothe inflamed airways. Parents should consider using a cool-mist humidifier in their child's room, particularly during nighttime, when symptoms may worsen. Additionally, keeping the child calm and well-hydrated can help reduce anxiety and further irritation of the throat, contributing to a more comfortable recovery process.

It is also important for parents to recognize the connection between croup and seasonal allergies. Allergens such as pollen, dust mites, and pet dander can exacerbate respiratory symptoms and increase the likelihood of viral infections. By managing seasonal allergies through appropriate treatments and reducing exposure to allergens, parents can potentially reduce the frequency and severity of croup episodes in their children. This proactive approach can lead to better overall respiratory health and fewer emergency situations.

Finally, understanding the long-term effects of recurrent croup is crucial for parents. Some children may experience multiple episodes of croup, which can lead to anxiety about future occurrences and an increased risk of developing other respiratory issues. Parents should educate themselves about the signs of croup in infants, as younger children may exhibit different symptoms compared to older children. By recognizing these symptoms early and implementing effective management strategies, parents can help their children navigate the challenges of croup and maintain a healthier respiratory system.

Prevention Strategies

Prevention strategies for croup focus on minimizing risk factors and managing symptoms effectively to reduce the frequency and severity of episodes. One of the most effective ways to prevent croup is to promote good hygiene practices among children. Teaching children the importance of regular handwashing, especially before meals and after being outside, can significantly decrease the likelihood of viral infections that lead to croup. Additionally, keeping children away from those who are ill and limiting their exposure to crowded places during peak illness seasons can help lower the risk of contracting respiratory viruses.

Creating a healthy home environment is another essential prevention strategy. Maintaining indoor air quality is crucial, as allergens such as dust, pet dander, and mold can exacerbate respiratory issues, including croup. Regularly cleaning and vacuuming your home, using air purifiers, and ensuring proper ventilation can help reduce these allergens. Furthermore, seasonal allergies can contribute to respiratory distress, so managing these allergies through appropriate treatments and avoiding known triggers will support overall respiratory health.

Utilizing humidifiers can also play a vital role in preventing croup symptoms, particularly during dry winter months. Humidifiers add moisture to the air, which can soothe irritated airways and help prevent the onset of croup. Parents should aim to keep humidity levels between 30% and 50% to maintain comfort without promoting mold growth. Additionally, steam inhalation can be beneficial; running a hot shower and allowing your child to breathe in the steam can provide relief from nasal congestion and throat irritation, reducing the likelihood of croup episodes.

It is important for parents to recognize signs of respiratory distress early on, as timely intervention can prevent the progression to more severe symptoms. Monitoring your child's breathing patterns and being aware of any changes can help you distinguish between croup and other respiratory illnesses. Keeping a close watch on your child's health during viral season, while being prepared to respond to symptoms promptly, can significantly impact the management of croup. If you notice persistent coughing, stridor, or difficulty breathing, seeking medical advice promptly can lead to early treatment and prevent complications.

Lastly, understanding the long-term effects of recurrent croup can guide parents in making informed decisions about prevention and treatment. While many children outgrow croup by the age of six, recurrent episodes can lead to ongoing respiratory issues or increased sensitivity to allergens. Parents should engage in regular discussions with healthcare providers about their child's health history and any recurrent symptoms. By implementing these prevention strategies and being proactive in managing your child's health, you can help reduce the frequency and severity of croup episodes, ensuring a healthier environment for your child.

Chapter 4: Home Remedies for Croup in Children

Natural Soothing Techniques

Natural soothing techniques can play a vital role in alleviating the discomfort associated with croup in children. Croup, characterized by a barking cough and stridor, often worsens at night and can be distressing for both the child and the parents. Understanding how to use natural remedies effectively can provide relief and comfort, minimizing the need for medical interventions. Parents can implement several approaches at home that not only target the symptoms of croup but also promote overall respiratory health.

One of the most effective natural treatments is the use of humidifiers. Moist air can soothe inflamed airways and ease breathing difficulties. A cool-mist humidifier placed in the child's room can help to reduce the severity of coughing spells and improve sleep quality. Regularly cleaning the humidifier is essential to prevent mold and bacteria buildup, which could exacerbate respiratory issues. Additionally, sitting with your child in a steamy bathroom while running a hot shower can provide immediate relief by allowing them to inhale warm, moist air.

Another natural approach involves the use of honey, which can be particularly effective for children over one year of age. Honey has soothing properties that can coat the throat and reduce coughing. Mixing honey with warm water or herbal tea can create a comforting drink that not only hydrates but also alleviates irritation. It is important to avoid honey for infants under one year due to the risk of botulism, a serious illness caused by bacteria that can thrive in honey.

Essential oils, when used carefully, can also offer soothing effects. Oils such as eucalyptus or lavender can be beneficial for their anti-inflammatory and calming properties. These can be diffused in the child's room or diluted with a carrier oil and applied to the chest for respiratory support. However, parents should always conduct a patch test before using any new essential oil on their child's skin and consult a pediatrician if there are concerns regarding allergies or sensitivities.

Lastly, maintaining a calm environment is crucial for managing croup symptoms. Stress and anxiety can worsen breathing difficulties, so creating a peaceful atmosphere can help soothe the child. Techniques such as gentle rocking, reading a favorite story, or playing soft music can promote relaxation. Additionally, ensuring that the child stays well-hydrated can support their immune system and aid recovery. By employing these natural soothing techniques, parents can provide comfort and relief during croup episodes while fostering a supportive environment for their child's healing process.

Effective At-Home Treatments

Effective at-home treatments for croup can significantly alleviate symptoms and provide comfort to children experiencing this viral respiratory illness. Croup is characterized by a distinctive barking cough, hoarseness, and difficulty breathing, often exacerbated by seasonal allergies. Parents can employ various home remedies to manage these symptoms effectively while ensuring their child's comfort and safety.

One of the most beneficial at-home treatments for croup is the use of a humidifier. Humidifiers add moisture to the air, which can soothe inflamed airways and reduce coughing fits, particularly during dry winter months when the air is less humid. It is essential to maintain the humidifier's cleanliness to prevent mold growth, which could worsen respiratory symptoms. If a humidifier is not available, taking the child into a bathroom filled with steam from a hot shower can have similar effects.

In addition to humidity, keeping the child well-hydrated is crucial. Encouraging the child to drink fluids can help thin mucus and keep the throat moist, which may ease coughing. Warm liquids, such as herbal teas or broth, can be particularly comforting. Parents should monitor their child's fluid intake and ensure they are drinking enough, as hydration plays a vital role in recovery and comfort.

Natural treatments can also be beneficial in managing croup symptoms. Honey is often recommended for children over one year old due to its soothing properties. A teaspoon of honey can help coat the throat and reduce coughing. Additionally, some parents find that essential oils like eucalyptus or lavender, when used in a diffuser, can promote relaxation and improve breathing. It is important, however, to consult a healthcare professional before trying any new treatment, particularly for younger children.

Finally, parents should be aware of the signs of severe croup or complications, as well as when to seek emergency treatment. Severe croup can cause significant breathing difficulties, stridor, or a bluish tint to the lips or face. While most cases of croup can be managed at home, understanding when to escalate care is crucial for ensuring the child's safety. By combining effective at-home treatments with vigilant monitoring, parents can help their children navigate the challenges of croup while minimizing discomfort and promoting recovery.

When to Seek Medical Attention

When managing a child's croup, it is crucial for parents to recognize the signs that indicate the need for medical attention. Croup typically presents with a distinctive bark-like cough, hoarseness, and stridor, which is a high-pitched wheezing sound during inhalation. While many cases of croup can be managed at home, there are specific symptoms that warrant immediate medical evaluation. If your child exhibits difficulty breathing, persistent stridor at rest, or if their lips or face develop a bluish tint, seek emergency care. These symptoms suggest that your child may be experiencing severe airway obstruction, requiring professional intervention.

Parents should also be vigilant about the overall severity of their child's symptoms. If the cough becomes increasingly severe and is accompanied by high fever, lethargy, or difficulty swallowing, it may indicate a more serious underlying infection. Viral infections are often the root cause of croup, but bacterial infections can also occur and may require antibiotics. If your child has croup and appears unusually tired or is not responding normally, it is essential to consult a healthcare provider to rule out any complications.

In infants, croup can be particularly concerning. If a baby under six months old displays symptoms of croup, parents should seek medical advice promptly. Infants are more vulnerable to respiratory distress, and their inability to communicate discomfort makes it imperative for parents to err on the side of caution. Additional signs to watch for in infants include rapid breathing, nasal flaring, or grunting sounds, all of which indicate the need for urgent medical assessment.

It is important to remember that while home remedies and natural treatments can alleviate mild croup symptoms, they are not substitutes for professional medical care in severe cases. Utilizing a humidifier can provide relief by adding moisture to the air, but if your child shows signs of significant distress, it is time to prioritize medical intervention. Home treatments are best suited for mild cases of croup, where parents can effectively manage symptoms with supportive care.

Finally, understanding the long-term implications of recurrent croup episodes is essential for parents. While most children outgrow croup by the age of five, recurring episodes may indicate an underlying issue, such as chronic allergies or other respiratory conditions. If your child experiences frequent bouts of croup, discussing these occurrences with a pediatrician can help identify potential triggers and develop a comprehensive management plan. Regular follow-ups can ensure that any chronic issues are addressed promptly, safeguarding your child's health and wellbeing.

Chapter 5: Natural Treatments for Croup Symptoms

Herbal Remedies

Herbal remedies have gained popularity among parents seeking natural treatment options for managing croup symptoms in children. Croup, characterized by a distinctive barking cough, stridor, and difficulty breathing, often arises from viral infections, particularly during the fall and winter months. While conventional treatments such as corticosteroids and nebulized epinephrine are effective, many parents look to herbal remedies as complementary options. Understanding these remedies, their potential benefits, and their appropriate application can empower parents in managing their child's croup.

One of the most commonly recommended herbal remedies for croup is thyme. This herb possesses natural antimicrobial properties and can help soothe the throat, potentially alleviating coughing fits. Parents can prepare a simple thyme tea by steeping fresh or dried thyme leaves in hot water. Once cooled, this tea can be given to children in small amounts, ensuring it is safe and palatable. Additionally, thyme can also be found in various herbal cough syrups formulated specifically for children, providing a convenient option for busy parents.

Another beneficial herb is marshmallow root, known for its mucilaginous properties that help coat the throat and reduce irritation. This remedy can be particularly helpful when a child's cough is persistent and bothersome. Marshmallow root can be infused in hot water or taken in capsule form, but it's essential to consult with a healthcare provider to determine the appropriate dosage for young children. This herbal remedy not only helps with croup symptoms but may also provide relief for other respiratory issues, making it a versatile option in a parent's herbal arsenal.

Honey, while not an herb, is often included in discussions of natural remedies due to its soothing qualities. For children over one year of age, a teaspoon of honey can help coat the throat and reduce coughing. Honey also has natural antimicrobial properties, which may assist in combating the underlying viral infection. However, it is crucial to remember that honey should never be given to infants under one year due to the risk of botulism. Parents should always exercise caution and consult with a pediatrician before introducing any new remedy, especially for younger children.

In addition to these remedies, the use of humidifiers can significantly improve a child's comfort during croup episodes. Adding moisture to the air helps soothe inflamed airways and can alleviate the harsh, dry cough associated with croup. Parents should ensure that the humidifier is clean and functioning properly to prevent the growth of mold and bacteria. By combining herbal remedies with environmental adjustments like humidification, parents can create a supportive atmosphere for their children, helping to manage croup symptoms more effectively and potentially reducing the need for medical intervention.

Essential Oils and Their Uses

Essential oils have gained popularity as natural remedies for various ailments, including respiratory issues like croup. When used appropriately, they can offer soothing effects that may help alleviate some symptoms associated with croup and enhance overall well-being. Parents seeking to manage their children's croup symptoms can explore certain essential oils known for their therapeutic properties. Among these, eucalyptus, tea tree, and lavender oils are particularly noted for their potential benefits in promoting respiratory health and providing comfort during episodes of croup.

Eucalyptus oil is widely recognized for its ability to support respiratory function. It has anti-inflammatory properties that may help reduce swelling in the airways, making it easier for children to breathe. When diffused in the air or diluted and applied topically (always with a carrier oil), eucalyptus oil can create a calming atmosphere that may ease coughing and congestion. Parents should ensure that the oil is used in moderation and consult with a healthcare provider, especially for younger children, to determine the best approach for usage.

Tea tree oil is another essential oil that may provide relief for children suffering from croup. Known for its antimicrobial properties, tea tree oil can help combat potential infections that may exacerbate respiratory symptoms. When used in a steam inhalation method or added to a warm bath, tea tree oil may help clear nasal passages and promote easier breathing. However, it is crucial to remember that tea tree oil should never be ingested and must always be diluted before topical application to avoid skin irritation.

Lavender oil is celebrated for its calming effects, making it an excellent choice for children experiencing the distressing symptoms of croup. In addition to its soothing aroma, lavender oil has anti-inflammatory properties that may contribute to reducing throat irritation and promoting a sense of relaxation. Parents can use lavender oil in a diffuser or apply it gently to the child's pillow to create a peaceful environment conducive to sleep, which is vital for recovery during bouts of croup.

While essential oils can be beneficial, they should be viewed as complementary therapies rather than replacements for conventional medical treatments. Parents should monitor their child's symptoms closely and seek professional medical advice if symptoms worsen or do not improve with home remedies. Understanding the appropriate use of essential oils in conjunction with other management strategies, such as maintaining humidity levels in the home or using prescribed medications, can empower parents to create a supportive environment for their children during episodes of croup.

Dietary Considerations

Dietary considerations can play a significant role in managing croup and its symptoms, especially in children who are prone to respiratory infections and seasonal allergies. A well-balanced diet that supports the immune system may help reduce the frequency and severity of croup episodes. Parents should focus on incorporating a variety of fruits, vegetables, whole grains, and lean proteins into their child's meals. Foods rich in vitamins A, C, and E, as well as zinc and omega-3 fatty acids, are particularly beneficial for bolstering immune function and reducing inflammation.

Hydration is another critical aspect of dietary considerations when dealing with croup. Keeping a child well-hydrated can help thin mucus secretions, making it easier for them to breathe. Encourage children to drink plenty of fluids, such as water, herbal teas, and broths. Warm liquids can be especially soothing and may help alleviate throat discomfort associated with croup. Avoiding overly sugary or caffeinated beverages is essential, as these can lead to dehydration and may worsen symptoms.

In addition to hydration, parents should be mindful of potential food allergens that could exacerbate seasonal allergies and, consequently, croup symptoms. Common allergens such as dairy, eggs, peanuts, and gluten can provoke allergic reactions in some children, leading to increased mucus production and respiratory distress. Keeping a food diary to track any correlations between specific foods and croup episodes can be beneficial. Consulting with a pediatrician or an allergist can provide guidance on appropriate dietary adjustments.

Certain foods may also help reduce inflammation and support respiratory health. Incorporating foods that contain natural anti-inflammatory properties, such as garlic, ginger, turmeric, and fatty fish, may provide additional relief for children experiencing croup symptoms. Parents should consider preparing meals that include these ingredients, which can enhance overall health and potentially minimize the impact of viral infections that lead to croup.

Finally, it is essential to be aware of the relationship between diet and overall well-being. A healthy diet not only supports immune function but can also improve a child's energy levels and mood, which can be particularly important during illness. By prioritizing nutrition and hydration, parents can take proactive steps in managing croup, ensuring their child is better equipped to handle respiratory challenges and recover more quickly.

Chapter 6: Croup Management for Parents

Creating a Care Plan

Creating a care plan for a child experiencing croup is essential for managing symptoms effectively and ensuring their comfort. A care plan should begin with a thorough understanding of the condition, including its symptoms and potential triggers. Parents should monitor their child's respiratory health and be aware of signs such as a barking cough, stridor, and difficulty breathing. Recognizing these symptoms early can prevent worsening and guide parents in seeking appropriate care. It is also beneficial to keep a symptom diary detailing the frequency and severity of episodes, helping to identify patterns or seasonal influences linked to allergies and viral infections.

Natural treatments can play a crucial role in the care plan for croup. Home remedies such as steam inhalation and warm baths can provide immediate relief by soothing irritated airways. Additionally, parents should consider using a cool-mist humidifier in their child's room. This device adds moisture to the air, which can ease breathing and reduce coughing during the night. Keeping the child well-hydrated is also vital; fluids help thin mucus and keep the throat moist, which can alleviate discomfort. Parents should consult with healthcare professionals to explore safe and effective natural treatments that fit their child's specific needs.

Incorporating allergy management into the care plan is critical, especially if the child has a known history of allergies. Parents should identify and minimize exposure to allergens, such as pollen, dust mites, and pet dander, particularly during peak allergy seasons. This can involve regular cleaning of the home environment, using air purifiers, and ensuring that the child avoids outdoor activities when pollen counts are high. Understanding the connection between croup and seasonal allergies enables parents to better prepare and adapt their care strategies, ultimately reducing the frequency of croup episodes.

It is important for parents to differentiate croup from other respiratory illnesses. While croup is typically characterized by a distinct barking cough and stridor, other conditions such as asthma and bronchitis might present similar symptoms but require different management strategies. A clear understanding of these differences can help parents take appropriate actions and avoid unnecessary stress during illness. Regular consultations with a pediatrician can also provide clarity and reassurance regarding the diagnosis and management of respiratory issues.

Lastly, parents should be aware of the potential long-term effects of recurrent croup. While most children outgrow croup by age five, some may experience repeated episodes that can lead to a cycle of anxiety surrounding illness. This can impact their overall health and wellbeing. In severe cases, parents should know when to seek emergency treatment, particularly if their child exhibits signs of severe distress or difficulty breathing. Crafting a comprehensive care plan that incorporates symptom management, natural treatments, allergy considerations, and education about croup will empower parents and help them support their child's health effectively.

Monitoring Symptoms

Monitoring symptoms of croup is essential for parents to effectively manage their child's condition. Croup is characterized by a distinctive barking cough, stridor, and hoarseness, typically resulting from viral infections that cause inflammation in the upper airways. Understanding these symptoms can help parents differentiate croup from other respiratory illnesses, such as asthma or bronchitis, which may require different interventions. Keeping a close eye on the frequency and intensity of these symptoms will help parents gauge the severity of their child's condition and make informed decisions regarding home care or the need for medical intervention.

Parents should be vigilant in observing any changes in their child's breathing patterns, especially at night when symptoms can often worsen. Stridor, a high-pitched wheezing sound, may indicate that the airway is becoming increasingly compromised. Other symptoms to monitor include difficulty swallowing, excessive drooling, or changes in color, such as a bluish tint around the lips or fingertips. If these symptoms escalate, it is crucial for parents to seek immediate medical attention, as severe croup can lead to respiratory distress and necessitate emergency treatment options.

In addition to recognizing the acute symptoms of croup, parents should also take note of the overall frequency of croup episodes. Some children may experience recurrent bouts of croup, which can be tied to underlying factors such as seasonal allergies. Tracking these occurrences can help identify triggers and facilitate discussions with healthcare providers about long-term management strategies. Parents can benefit from keeping a symptom diary, noting the intensity of symptoms, any accompanying illnesses, and environmental factors that may contribute to flare-ups.

Home remedies and natural treatments can play an important role in managing mild croup symptoms. Utilizing a humidifier in the child's room can help soothe inflamed airways by adding moisture to the air, making it easier for the child to breathe. Additionally, steam inhalation, warm baths, and ensuring the child stays well-hydrated can alleviate discomfort. While these methods can offer relief, parents should remain aware of their child's condition and be prepared to seek further medical advice if symptoms do not improve or worsen over time.

Finally, understanding the long-term effects of recurrent croup is vital for parents to consider. Frequent episodes can lead to increased anxiety for both the child and the parents, and in some cases, may impact the child's overall respiratory health. By monitoring symptoms closely and maintaining open communication with healthcare providers, parents can create a proactive approach to managing croup and its related complications. This vigilance not only aids in immediate symptom control but also equips parents with the knowledge needed for future episodes, ultimately ensuring better health outcomes for their children.

Communicating with Healthcare Providers

Effective communication with healthcare providers is essential for parents managing croup in their children. When seeking medical advice, it is vital to clearly articulate symptoms and any changes observed in your child's condition. This includes detailing the onset of symptoms such as a barking cough, stridor, or difficulty breathing, as these indicators can help healthcare professionals assess the severity of the situation. Preparing for appointments by jotting down notes on your child's symptoms, medical history, and any home remedies or treatments you have tried can facilitate a more productive dialogue with your provider.

When discussing croup, parents should be prepared to ask specific questions about the condition. Inquire about the potential causes of croup, including its connection to viral infections and seasonal allergies. Understanding these connections can aid in comprehending how environmental factors might influence your child's health. Additionally, ask about the differences between croup and other respiratory illnesses, as this knowledge can help you gauge when to seek further medical intervention. Having a good grasp of these topics will empower you in conversations with healthcare professionals.

It is also essential to discuss treatment options with your provider. Parents might be interested in exploring natural treatments and home remedies for managing croup symptoms. Be open about any alternative therapies you are considering or currently using, such as humidifiers or saline nasal drops. These conversations can help healthcare providers offer tailored advice that aligns with your family's preferences while ensuring the safety and effectiveness of any treatments. They can also provide guidance on when to use emergency treatment options for severe croup, which is crucial for serious cases.

In addition to treatment discussions, parents should address any concerns about long-term effects of recurrent croup. While many children outgrow croup as they get older, understanding the potential implications for respiratory health is important. Healthcare providers can help clarify any misconceptions and offer strategies for managing recurrent episodes. This proactive approach allows parents to feel more equipped to handle future occurrences while fostering a collaborative relationship with their healthcare team.

Finally, parents should establish a rapport with their child's healthcare provider. Regular check-ups and open lines of communication can make a significant difference in managing croup and other respiratory issues. This relationship fosters trust, ensuring that parents feel comfortable seeking advice and sharing concerns as they arise. By being proactive in communication, parents can better navigate the complexities of croup management, access appropriate interventions, and ultimately enhance their child's well-being.

Chapter 7: The Role of Humidifiers in Treating Croup

Benefits of Humidified Air

Humidified air plays a crucial role in alleviating the symptoms of croup, particularly for young children who are susceptible to this respiratory condition. Croup is characterized by a distinctive barking cough, stridor, and hoarseness, which can be exacerbated by dry air. When humidity levels are increased, the moisture helps to soothe the inflamed tissues in the throat and airway, making it easier for children to breathe. This is especially important during the colder months when indoor heating can significantly lower humidity levels, aggravating respiratory issues.

One of the primary benefits of using a humidifier is its ability to reduce the severity of coughing fits associated with croup. The added moisture in the air helps to keep the airways hydrated, which can minimize irritation and reduce the frequency of coughing. Parents often observe a noticeable improvement in their child's comfort level when using a humidifier, as the moist air can help to ease the tightness in the chest and throat. This is particularly beneficial during night-time, when coughing can disrupt sleep for both the child and parents.

In addition to providing relief from croup symptoms, humidified air can also assist in managing seasonal allergies that often coincide with respiratory infections. Many allergens, such as pollen and dust mites, thrive in dry environments. By maintaining optimal humidity levels, parents can create a less hospitable environment for these allergens, thereby reducing the likelihood of allergic reactions in children. This dual benefit of addressing both croup and seasonal allergies makes humidifiers a valuable tool in a parent's arsenal for managing their child's health.

Furthermore, humidified air can be beneficial in preventing secondary infections that may complicate a child's health during episodes of croup. When airways are dry, they can become more susceptible to viruses and bacteria, leading to further respiratory illnesses. By keeping the airways moist, humidifiers can help to support the natural defense mechanisms of the respiratory system, potentially reducing the risk of developing additional infections. This aspect is particularly important for children who experience recurrent croup, as they are often more vulnerable to subsequent respiratory issues.

Lastly, using a humidifier is a simple, non-invasive remedy that parents can easily incorporate into their home care routines. While medical treatments may be necessary during severe episodes of croup, maintaining a humid environment can complement these interventions and promote overall respiratory health. Parents should ensure their humidifiers are well-maintained and clean to avoid the introduction of mold or bacteria into the air, which could counteract the benefits. By understanding and utilizing the advantages of humidified air, parents can play an active role in managing their child's croup symptoms and enhancing their overall well-being.

Choosing the Right Humidifier

Choosing the right humidifier is a crucial step for parents managing croup and its associated symptoms in children. Humidifiers work by adding moisture to the air, which can help soothe inflamed airways and alleviate coughing caused by viral infections. When selecting a humidifier, consider the type of humidifier, the size of the room, and the maintenance requirements. There are several types available, including cool mist, warm mist, and ultrasonic humidifiers, each with its unique benefits and drawbacks that can impact your child's comfort during croup episodes.

Cool mist humidifiers are often recommended for croup management because they can help lower air temperature while adding moisture, making breathing easier for children experiencing respiratory distress. On the other hand, warm mist humidifiers can create a comforting environment, especially during colder months, but they may pose a burn risk if not used carefully. Ultrasonic humidifiers are also a popular option due to their quiet operation and energy efficiency. Parents should assess their home environment to determine which type will best suit their needs and ensure the humidifier is safe for young children.

Room size is another important factor when choosing a humidifier. It's essential to select a model that is appropriate for the size of the room where your child sleeps or spends most of their time. A unit that is too small may not effectively increase humidity levels, while one that is too large could create excessive moisture, potentially leading to mold growth and other respiratory issues. Many manufacturers provide guidelines on room size compatibility, which can help parents make an informed decision.

Maintenance is key to ensuring the humidifier operates effectively and safely. Regular cleaning is necessary to prevent mold and bacteria buildup, which can exacerbate respiratory problems. Parents should follow the manufacturer's instructions for cleaning and changing water daily to ensure optimal performance. Some models come with features that make maintenance easier, such as dishwasher-safe parts or built-in filters, which can be beneficial for busy families managing the challenges of croup and seasonal allergies.

Lastly, while humidifiers can provide symptomatic relief, they should be part of a broader approach to managing croup and respiratory illnesses in children. Parents should also be aware of other home remedies and natural treatments that can complement the use of a humidifier, such as ensuring proper hydration, using saline nasal drops, and maintaining a smoke-free environment. By combining these strategies, parents can create a supportive atmosphere that promotes healing and comfort for their children when facing the discomfort of croup.

Best Practices for Humidifier Use

When using a humidifier to alleviate croup symptoms in children, it is essential to select the right type for your needs. Cool mist humidifiers are often recommended for croup treatment as they help to soothe inflamed airways and reduce respiratory distress. Avoid using warm mist humidifiers, as the heat can potentially worsen inflammation and pose a burn risk. Additionally, consider a humidifier with a built-in hygrometer that allows you to monitor humidity levels, ensuring they remain within the recommended range of 30-50 percent.

Proper placement of the humidifier is also crucial for maximizing its effectiveness. Position the device in your child's bedroom, ideally a few feet away from the bed, to allow for optimal mist distribution without overwhelming the space. Ensure the humidifier is placed on a sturdy surface where it won't tip over and away from any electronic devices. Regularly check that the mist is not directly blowing onto your child's face, as this can cause discomfort.

Regular maintenance of your humidifier is vital to prevent the growth of mold and bacteria, which can exacerbate respiratory issues. Clean the humidifier daily by emptying the water tank, rinsing it out, and wiping down surfaces with a soft cloth. Weekly, perform a more thorough cleaning using a mixture of vinegar and water or a manufacturer-recommended solution to eliminate any buildup. Always refer to the user manual for specific cleaning guidelines to ensure the longevity and safety of your device.

In addition to using a humidifier, consider creating a comfortable environment that supports your child's recovery. Keep the room well-ventilated and avoid exposing your child to tobacco smoke or other irritants that could aggravate croup symptoms. Dress your child in lightweight clothing to prevent overheating, as excessive warmth can worsen respiratory discomfort. Encourage your child to drink plenty of fluids to stay hydrated, as this can help thin mucus and ease breathing.

Lastly, monitor your child's symptoms closely while using a humidifier. If you notice a sudden worsening of symptoms, such as difficulty breathing or stridor, seek medical attention immediately. While humidifiers can provide significant relief, they are not a substitute for professional medical advice or treatment. Ensure you have a plan in place for emergencies, and maintain open communication with your pediatrician about your child's condition and any concerns you may have during their recovery from croup.

Chapter 8: Croup vs. Other Respiratory Illnesses

Differentiating Croup from Other Conditions

Croup is a common respiratory condition in children characterized by a distinctive barking cough, often accompanied by stridor and respiratory distress. However, differentiating croup from other similar respiratory illnesses is crucial for effective management and treatment. Common conditions that may mimic croup include viral laryngitis, bronchitis, and asthma. Each of these conditions presents with overlapping symptoms but requires different approaches to treatment and care. Parents should be aware of these distinctions to ensure their child receives appropriate care.

Viral laryngitis is often confused with croup due to the similar inflammation in the larynx. Children with viral laryngitis typically exhibit a hoarse voice and mild fever but do not usually experience the severe barking cough associated with croup. In contrast, the cough in croup is more pronounced and is often worse at night. Recognizing these differences can help parents determine whether to manage symptoms at home or seek medical attention, especially if symptoms worsen or do not improve.

Bronchitis, another respiratory condition, may lead to a persistent cough and wheezing. While both conditions can occur following a viral infection, bronchitis is primarily associated with inflammation in the bronchi rather than the larynx. Parents should look for additional symptoms such as increased mucus production and chest discomfort, which are more indicative of bronchitis than croup. Understanding these nuances can assist in identifying when to consult a healthcare provider for further evaluation.

Asthma can also present with cough and respiratory distress, particularly in children with a history of wheezing or allergic reactions. Unlike croup, asthma is typically characterized by a more chronic cough and can be triggered by allergens, exercise, or respiratory infections. It is essential for parents to monitor their child's symptoms closely and recognize patterns that may suggest asthma rather than croup, especially if there is a family history of asthma or allergies.

Finally, it is important for parents to be aware of the potential for other respiratory infections that can complicate or resemble croup. Conditions such as epiglottitis, which is a medical emergency, can present with severe respiratory distress, high fever, and drooling. Parents should seek immediate medical attention if they notice these symptoms. By understanding the differences between croup and other respiratory illnesses, parents can take proactive steps in managing their child's health and ensuring timely interventions when necessary.

Similar Symptoms and How to Tell Them Apart

Croup is often mistaken for other respiratory illnesses due to overlapping symptoms. The hallmark of croup is a distinct "barking" cough, usually accompanied by a hoarse voice and stridor, which is a high-pitched wheezing sound occurring during inhalation. However, these symptoms can also present in conditions such as bronchitis, asthma, or even allergic reactions. Parents should be vigilant in observing the specific characteristics of their child's cough and breathing patterns to differentiate croup from other ailments.

When assessing whether a child's symptoms align with croup, it is essential to note the context. Croup is most commonly caused by viral infections, particularly parainfluenza viruses, and typically occurs in children aged six months to three years. In contrast, bronchitis may follow a cold and can be associated with mucus production, while asthma often features wheezing and difficulty exhaling, which may not be as pronounced in croup. Understanding these nuances can help parents identify the illness more accurately, leading to appropriate management strategies.

Seasonal allergies can also mimic some symptoms of croup, leading to confusion among parents. Allergic reactions may cause coughing, throat irritation, and nasal congestion, but they usually lack the characteristic barking cough and stridor associated with croup. In cases of seasonal allergies, children often exhibit sneezing and watery eyes, which are not typical in croup episodes. Parents should consider environmental triggers and their child's allergic history when evaluating symptoms, as this may guide them toward the right treatment approach.

Another condition to consider is epiglottitis, a serious bacterial infection that can lead to airway obstruction. While epiglottitis is less common due to widespread vaccination against Haemophilus influenzae type b, it can present with a sudden onset of high fever, drooling, and severe difficulty breathing. Unlike croup, which develops gradually over a few days, epiglottitis can escalate rapidly and requires immediate medical attention. Parents should be aware of these critical differences and seek emergency care if they suspect epiglottitis.

In managing croup, parents can utilize natural treatments and home remedies to alleviate symptoms, such as using a humidifier to moisten the air, which can help soothe the throat and reduce coughing. However, if a child exhibits severe symptoms—such as difficulty breathing, stridor at rest, or extreme lethargy—emergency treatment options, including corticosteroids or nebulized epinephrine, may be necessary. By understanding the similarities and differences between croup and other respiratory illnesses, parents can make informed decisions regarding their child's health and well-being.

When to Visit the Doctor

When it comes to croup, understanding when to seek medical attention is crucial for the well-being of your child. Croup typically presents with a distinctive barking cough, hoarseness, and difficulty breathing, symptoms that can escalate quickly. Parents should be vigilant and monitor their child's condition closely, particularly during the night when symptoms may worsen. If your child exhibits signs of significant respiratory distress, such as stridor (a high-pitched wheezing sound), retractions (pulling in of the chest muscles), or rapid breathing, it is essential to consult a healthcare professional immediately.

In addition to respiratory distress, parents should be mindful of other concerning symptoms that may indicate the need for a doctor's visit. If your child has a high fever that persists despite the use of fever-reducing medications, or if they appear unusually lethargic or irritable, these could be warning signs of a more serious infection. Persistent symptoms lasting longer than three to five days, or a sudden worsening of their condition, should also prompt a visit to the pediatrician. It is always better to err on the side of caution, as prompt medical evaluation can prevent complications from developing.

For parents managing croup at home, it is essential to recognize what constitutes severe croup. If your child is unable to drink fluids due to difficulty swallowing or if they show signs of dehydration, medical assistance is necessary. Moreover, if your child's symptoms do not improve with home remedies such as humidifiers, steam inhalation, or natural treatments, seeking medical advice is advisable. In some cases, prescription medications such as corticosteroids may be required to reduce inflammation and alleviate symptoms effectively.

Understanding the connection between croup and seasonal allergies can also inform parents when deciding to seek medical help. Allergies can exacerbate respiratory symptoms, and if a child with croup is also experiencing allergy flare-ups, the combination may lead to increased difficulty in breathing. Monitoring for allergy-related symptoms like nasal congestion or sneezing, along with croup symptoms, can help parents make informed decisions about whether to visit their healthcare provider.

Finally, it is important for parents to be aware of the long-term effects of recurrent croup and to keep an open line of communication with their child's healthcare provider. Children who experience multiple episodes of croup may be at risk for developing asthma or other respiratory conditions later in life. Regular check-ups can help manage and monitor these risks, ensuring that your child receives appropriate care and support. If you have any concerns about your child's respiratory health or the frequency of croup episodes, do not hesitate to reach out to your doctor for guidance.

Chapter 9: Long-Term Effects of Recurrent Croup

Understanding Recurrence

Recurrence is a critical aspect of croup that every parent should understand, especially since many children experience multiple episodes throughout their early years. Croup, primarily caused by viral infections, often manifests as a barking cough, hoarseness, and difficulty breathing due to airway inflammation. The viral pathogens responsible for croup, such as the parainfluenza virus, are prevalent among young children, making recurrent episodes common. Parents should be aware that once a child has experienced croup, their susceptibility to future episodes may be heightened, especially during the fall and winter months when respiratory viruses circulate more widely.

One significant factor contributing to the recurrence of croup is the connection between viral infections and seasonal allergies. Many children who suffer from croup also have underlying allergies, which can aggravate their respiratory system and make them more prone to airway inflammation. Parents should monitor their children's allergy symptoms closely, as managing these can help reduce the frequency and severity of croup episodes. This might include employing natural treatments such as saline nasal sprays and ensuring that the home environment is free of allergens that could trigger respiratory issues.

Another essential consideration is the role of humidifiers in managing croup symptoms. Dry air can exacerbate the inflammation in a child's airway, leading to a higher likelihood of repeated croup episodes. Using a cool-mist humidifier in the child's bedroom can add moisture to the air, providing relief from the symptoms of croup and potentially preventing recurrence. Alongside this, other home remedies like warm baths or steam inhalation can also be beneficial in soothing the child's throat and easing their breathing.

Parents should also differentiate croup from other respiratory illnesses such as asthma or bronchitis, as the management strategies may differ significantly. Understanding these differences is crucial for parents in recognizing when their child requires medical attention. While croup is often manageable at home, severe cases may lead to complications that necessitate emergency treatment options. Parents should be equipped with knowledge regarding the signs of severe croup, such as stridor at rest or significant difficulty breathing, so they can act quickly to ensure their child's safety.

Finally, it's important to consider the long-term effects of recurrent croup episodes on a child's respiratory health. Although many children outgrow croup by age six, recurrent infections can potentially lead to lasting respiratory issues. Parents should maintain open communication with their pediatrician to track their child's health and address any ongoing concerns. By understanding the patterns of croup recurrence and its management, parents can better support their children through these challenging episodes and promote their overall well-being.

Potential Complications

Potential complications of croup can vary significantly depending on the severity of the condition and the age of the child. While most cases of croup are mild and manageable at home, it is crucial for parents to be aware of potential complications that may arise. One of the most concerning complications is the risk of respiratory distress. This occurs when the swelling in the airways becomes severe enough to hinder normal breathing. Children with underlying respiratory issues, such as asthma, may be at a higher risk for experiencing significant complications, making it imperative for parents to monitor their child's symptoms closely.

Another potential complication is the development of secondary bacterial infections. While croup is primarily caused by viral infections, the inflammation and irritation in the throat can create an environment conducive to bacterial growth. Parents should be vigilant for signs of secondary infections, such as persistent fever, increased cough, or a change in the character of the cough, as these can indicate the need for medical evaluation and possible antibiotic treatment. Recognizing these signs early can help prevent more severe health issues.

In some cases, recurrent episodes of croup can lead to long-term effects, especially in young children. Frequent bouts of croup may result in an increased sensitivity of the airways, making a child more susceptible to respiratory illnesses later in life. Additionally, children with recurrent croup may experience anxiety or stress associated with the symptoms and their management, potentially affecting their overall well-being. Parents should be aware of these long-term implications and consider discussing them with their pediatrician if their child experiences multiple episodes.

When managing croup, parents should also be cautious about the use of home remedies. While many natural treatments, such as honey or warm fluids, can provide symptom relief, there is a risk of inadvertently overlooking more serious symptoms that require medical attention. Furthermore, not all home remedies are appropriate for all ages, especially infants. Parents should be informed about safe practices and consult healthcare professionals before implementing any new treatment strategies, ensuring that they are addressing the condition appropriately without compromising their child's health.

Finally, severe cases of croup may necessitate emergency treatment options. Parents must be prepared to recognize when a child's symptoms escalate beyond what can be managed at home. Signs such as stridor at rest, severe difficulty breathing, or cyanosis indicate an urgent need for medical intervention. Understanding the timeline for when to seek help and knowing the available emergency options can significantly impact outcomes. By staying informed and attentive, parents can navigate the complexities of croup management effectively, minimizing potential complications while ensuring their child's safety.

Strategies for Reducing Recurrences

To effectively manage croup and reduce its recurrence in children, parents can implement several proactive strategies. One of the most critical steps is to maintain a healthy environment that minimizes exposure to common viral infections, which are significant triggers for croup. Regular handwashing, encouraging children to avoid close contact with sick peers, and ensuring that their vaccinations are up to date can significantly reduce the likelihood of viral infections that lead to croup. Additionally, teaching children proper respiratory hygiene, such as covering their mouths when coughing or sneezing, can further help limit the spread of germs.

Utilizing humidifiers in your child's room can also play a vital role in managing croup symptoms and preventing recurrences. Dry air can exacerbate respiratory issues, making it essential to maintain an optimal humidity level. A cool mist humidifier can help soothe the throat and nasal passages, reducing inflammation and discomfort. Parents should ensure that humidifiers are regularly cleaned to prevent the growth of mold and bacteria, which can worsen respiratory symptoms. In addition, steamy baths or showers can provide immediate relief during croup episodes and create a more comfortable environment.

Natural treatments and home remedies can further support your child's recovery and help prevent future episodes of croup. Honey, for instance, is known for its soothing properties and can be given to children over one year of age to alleviate throat discomfort. Herbal remedies, such as chamomile tea, may also provide relief due to their anti-inflammatory properties. Always consult with a healthcare provider before introducing any new treatments to ensure they are safe and appropriate for your child's age and health status.

Recognizing the connection between seasonal allergies and croup is crucial for parents. Allergies can contribute to respiratory inflammation, making children more susceptible to croup. Implementing strategies to manage seasonal allergies, such as using air purifiers, keeping windows closed during high pollen seasons, and regularly cleaning your home to reduce dust and allergens, can help create a healthier environment. Allergy medications may also be beneficial, but parents should discuss these options with their child's pediatrician for personalized advice.

Lastly, understanding the signs of severe croup is essential for timely intervention. Parents should be aware of symptoms such as stridor (a high-pitched wheezing sound), difficulty breathing, or a rapid heartbeat. If these symptoms appear, emergency treatment options, such as corticosteroids or nebulized epinephrine, may be necessary. Educating yourself about croup and its management will empower parents to take proactive steps in reducing recurrences and ensuring the well-being of their children.

Chapter 10: Croup in Infants: Signs and Care Tips

Identifying Croup in Infants

Identifying croup in infants is crucial for prompt management and comfort. Croup typically emerges following a viral infection, and its hallmark symptom is a distinctive cough that resembles the sound of a barking seal. In infants, this cough may be accompanied by stridor, a high-pitched wheezing sound that occurs during inhalation. Parents should also be attentive to changes in their infant's breathing patterns, as labored or rapid breathing can indicate that the condition is worsening. Observing these symptoms early can help in determining the severity of croup and the need for intervention.

In addition to the barking cough and stridor, other signs of croup in infants may include a hoarse voice, difficulty swallowing, and a general sense of distress or agitation. Infants may become more irritable than usual, often due to discomfort or difficulty breathing. Parents should monitor their child's temperature, as fevers can accompany viral infections that lead to croup. It is essential to remain calm and assess the situation as accurately as possible, as the symptoms can sometimes escalate quickly.

Croup symptoms may worsen at night, making it essential for parents to be vigilant during evening hours. If an infant's breathing becomes increasingly labored, or if they show signs of cyanosis—bluish discoloration of the lips or face—immediate medical attention is critical. Understanding the timeline of symptoms can also help parents gauge whether the condition is improving or deteriorating. Croup often lasts for several days, with symptoms typically peaking around the second or third day.

Home remedies can provide relief for infants suffering from croup. Using a humidifier in the infant's room can help maintain moisture in the air, which may ease breathing difficulties. Additionally, keeping the child calm, as crying can exacerbate breathing issues, is important. Parents should also consider elevating the infant's head while sleeping to promote easier breathing. Natural treatments, such as honey for children over one year old, can soothe the throat, although this should be avoided in younger infants due to the risk of botulism.

Understanding the connection between croup and seasonal allergies is also important for parents. Allergies can exacerbate respiratory conditions, making it more likely for infants to experience croup following exposure to allergens. Knowledge of the signs of croup, how to manage symptoms, and when to seek emergency treatment can empower parents to effectively care for their infants. By staying informed and prepared, parents can navigate the challenges of croup and provide relief for their little ones during this distressing time.

Safe Care Practices

Safe care practices are essential for parents managing croup in their children, especially during peak seasons when respiratory illnesses are prevalent. Croup, characterized by a distinctive cough and difficulty breathing, can be distressing for both children and parents. By understanding and implementing safe care practices, parents can better navigate the challenges of this condition. This includes recognizing the signs of croup, knowing when to seek medical help, and being aware of effective home remedies that can alleviate symptoms.

One of the primary safe care practices is monitoring your child's symptoms closely. Parents should familiarize themselves with the typical signs of croup, which often include a harsh, barking cough, hoarseness, and stridor, a high-pitched wheezing sound during breathing. Keeping a close eye on these symptoms will enable parents to determine the severity of the condition. If symptoms worsen or if the child displays signs of severe difficulty breathing, such as retractions (where the skin pulls in around the ribs and neck), immediate medical attention is necessary.

In addition to monitoring symptoms, parents can implement various home remedies to provide relief. Using a humidifier in the child's room can significantly ease breathing difficulties. Humidifiers add moisture to the air, which can soothe the inflamed airways. Furthermore, parents may find that taking the child into a steamy bathroom or stepping outside for fresh, cool air can also help alleviate symptoms. These practices are not only safe but can also provide comfort to the child during episodes of croup.

It is important for parents to understand the role of seasonal allergies in croup. Allergens such as pollen and dust mites can exacerbate respiratory issues, making it crucial to maintain a clean and allergen-free environment. Regular cleaning, using air purifiers, and ensuring that the child's bedding is free of dust can contribute to a healthier atmosphere. Awareness of these connections will empower parents to take proactive steps in managing both croup and seasonal allergies, ultimately leading to a better quality of life for their children.

Finally, parents should be informed about emergency treatment options for severe cases of croup. In some instances, a healthcare provider may recommend corticosteroids to reduce inflammation in the airways. Recognizing when to utilize these options is vital for safe care practices. Parents should have a plan in place for emergencies, including knowing the nearest medical facility and having a list of symptoms that warrant immediate intervention. By combining knowledge of safe care practices with awareness of treatment options, parents can effectively manage croup and ensure the well-being of their children.

When to Seek Urgent Care

When dealing with croup, it is essential for parents to recognize when their child's condition requires urgent care. Croup is often characterized by a distinctive barking cough, hoarseness, and stridor, but not all cases will respond to home remedies or natural treatments. Parents should monitor the severity of symptoms carefully. If your child exhibits signs of respiratory distress, such as difficulty breathing, rapid or labored breathing, or a noticeable change in their skin color, it is crucial to seek medical attention immediately. These symptoms may indicate that the airway is becoming obstructed or that the child is experiencing a more severe form of croup, which necessitates prompt evaluation by healthcare professionals.

In addition to respiratory distress, parents should be vigilant for signs of dehydration, which can occur if a child is unable to drink fluids due to throat swelling or pain. Symptoms of dehydration include dry mouth, decreased urination, and lethargy. If your child shows these signs, it is vital to contact a healthcare provider without delay. In some cases, children may require intravenous fluids or other interventions to ensure they remain hydrated and stable. Understanding the signs of dehydration and being proactive can prevent further complications.

Fever is another critical factor to consider when assessing your child's condition. A high fever, especially one that persists despite the use of fever-reducing medications, can indicate a more serious underlying infection. When croup is accompanied by a high fever that does not respond to treatment, parents should not hesitate to consult a physician. This can help rule out other viral infections that might mimic croup but require different management strategies. Timely evaluation can lead to appropriate medical interventions that may alleviate the child's symptoms more effectively.

It's also important to recognize when croup symptoms do not improve with standard home management techniques, such as the use of humidifiers or natural remedies. If your child's symptoms worsen or do not show signs of improvement within a few days, it may be time to seek urgent care. Persistent symptoms can be a sign of a more severe infection or the potential for recurrent croup, which may require additional medical evaluation and intervention. Parents should trust their instincts and seek care if they feel their child is not improving.

Lastly, for infants, the signs of croup can sometimes be less obvious, making it even more crucial for parents to be attentive and informed. If an infant shows symptoms of croup, such as a barking cough or difficulty breathing, immediate medical attention is warranted. Infants are particularly vulnerable, and their small airways can become obstructed more quickly than in older children. Ensuring that you are aware of the signs and when to seek urgent care can help manage your child's health effectively and prevent long-term complications associated with recurrent croup or other respiratory illnesses.

Chapter 11: Emergency Treatment Options for Severe Croup

Recognizing Severe Croup Symptoms

Recognizing severe croup symptoms is crucial for parents to ensure timely intervention and effective management. Croup typically presents with a distinctive barking cough, which can often escalate in severity. In cases of severe croup, the cough may become more pronounced, accompanied by stridor, a high-pitched wheezing sound that occurs during inhalation. This stridor is a key indicator of airway narrowing and signifies that the child may be struggling to breathe effectively. It's essential for parents to monitor the severity of these symptoms, as they often indicate the need for immediate medical attention.

In addition to the barking cough and stridor, parents should be vigilant for signs of respiratory distress, such as rapid breathing, retractions (the sinking of the skin between the ribs or around the collarbone during inhalation), and difficulty speaking or crying due to shortness of breath. Children may also exhibit changes in their skin color, particularly around the lips or face, which can signify inadequate oxygenation. Recognizing these alarming signs early can lead to quicker responses and interventions that can significantly improve outcomes.

Another symptom that may accompany severe croup is a high fever. While mild fever can be common with viral infections, a temperature above 102°F (39°C) can indicate a more intense illness and may exacerbate symptoms. Parents should also pay attention to their child's overall behavior; lethargy and irritability can be signs of distress and warrant further evaluation. It is important to note that while some symptoms may appear mild at first, they can rapidly progress to more severe forms, making it essential for parents to stay alert and proactive.

The connection between croup and seasonal allergies is also noteworthy. Allergic reactions can sometimes exacerbate respiratory symptoms, leading to increased inflammation in the airways. Parents should be aware that if their child has a history of allergies, the onset of croup symptoms might be influenced by their allergic status. Keeping a close eye on environmental triggers and managing allergies can help reduce the frequency and severity of croup episodes, allowing for better overall respiratory health.

In severe cases, emergency treatment options may become necessary, including corticosteroids or nebulized epinephrine to reduce airway swelling. Parents must be aware of when to seek emergency care, especially if their child exhibits severe symptoms such as significant difficulty breathing, persistent stridor at rest, or extreme lethargy. Understanding these severe symptoms empowers parents to act quickly and effectively, ensuring their child's safety and well-being during a potentially frightening episode of croup.

At-Home Emergency Measures

At-home emergency measures play a crucial role in managing croup symptoms effectively, allowing parents to provide immediate relief to their children. The first step in addressing croup is to recognize its symptoms, which often include a distinctive barking cough, stridor, and difficulty breathing. If your child exhibits these signs, it's essential to stay calm and assess the severity of their condition. Mild cases can often be managed at home, but if your child is experiencing significant breathing difficulties, high fever, or lethargy, it is vital to seek medical attention promptly.

Creating a comfortable environment is key to alleviating the distress caused by croup. One effective method is to use a humidifier in your child's room. Humidifiers add moisture to the air, which can help soothe inflamed airways and reduce coughing. Make sure to keep the humidifier clean to prevent the growth of mold and bacteria, which could worsen respiratory issues. Alternatively, if a humidifier is unavailable, sitting in a steamy bathroom with your child can provide similar relief. The warm, moist air can help ease their breathing and soothe their throat.

In addition to humidity, staying hydrated is essential for children suffering from croup. Encourage your child to drink plenty of fluids, as staying hydrated can help thin mucus secretions, making it easier for them to breathe. Warm fluids, such as broth or herbal tea, can be particularly soothing. If your child is very young or reluctant to drink, consider offering ice chips or popsicles, which can provide hydration while also soothing their throat.

Some parents find that natural remedies can complement traditional treatments for croup. Honey, for example, is known for its soothing properties and can help alleviate throat irritation. However, honey should only be given to children over one year of age due to the risk of botulism in infants. Additionally, maintaining a calm environment and using distraction techniques, such as reading a book or watching a favorite movie, can help reduce anxiety and make it easier for your child to cope with their symptoms.

Monitoring your child's condition is crucial during a croup episode. Keep an eye on their breathing pattern, and watch for any signs of worsening symptoms. If your child's stridor becomes more pronounced, or if they have difficulty speaking or swallowing, it may indicate a more severe case of croup. In such situations, emergency treatments, such as corticosteroids or nebulized epinephrine, may be necessary, and contacting a healthcare provider is imperative. Understanding these at-home emergency measures can empower parents to provide immediate care and ensure their child receives the appropriate treatment when needed.

Professional Medical Interventions

Professional medical interventions for croup are essential to understand, particularly for parents managing their child's health. While many cases of croup are mild and can be effectively treated at home, there are instances where professional care is necessary to ensure the child's safety and comfort. Medical interventions typically involve a thorough assessment by a healthcare professional, who will evaluate the severity of the croup based on the child's symptoms and overall condition. Key indicators for seeking medical help include difficulty breathing, stridor at rest, lethargy, or signs of dehydration.

In cases where croup is moderate to severe, healthcare providers may recommend corticosteroids to reduce airway inflammation. Dexamethasone is commonly used due to its efficacy and ease of administration. This medication helps alleviate symptoms and speeds up recovery, making it a cornerstone of medical treatment for croup. In addition to corticosteroids, nebulized epinephrine may be administered in a clinical setting for immediate relief of airway swelling. This intervention can provide rapid improvement in breathing, particularly in more severe cases.

Another critical aspect of professional medical interventions involves the use of supportive care. Oxygen therapy may be necessary if the child exhibits signs of respiratory distress or low oxygen saturation levels. This intervention ensures that the child receives adequate oxygen supply while the underlying condition is being treated. In some instances, hospitalization may be required for close monitoring and more intensive treatment, especially in young infants or children with underlying health issues.

Parents should also be aware of the potential need for further diagnostic evaluations if recurrent croup is a concern. Healthcare providers may recommend tests to rule out other underlying conditions, such as allergies or anatomical abnormalities that could contribute to recurrent episodes. Understanding these factors can help parents manage their child's health more effectively and make informed decisions about treatment options.

Finally, it's important for parents to maintain open communication with healthcare professionals regarding their child's symptoms and responses to treatment. Keeping a detailed record of episodes, including triggers and severity, can aid in discussions with healthcare providers. By understanding the role of professional medical interventions, parents can be better equipped to navigate the complexities of croup and ensure their child's well-being during episodes of respiratory distress.